RESTORATIVE YOGA

FOR SENIORS

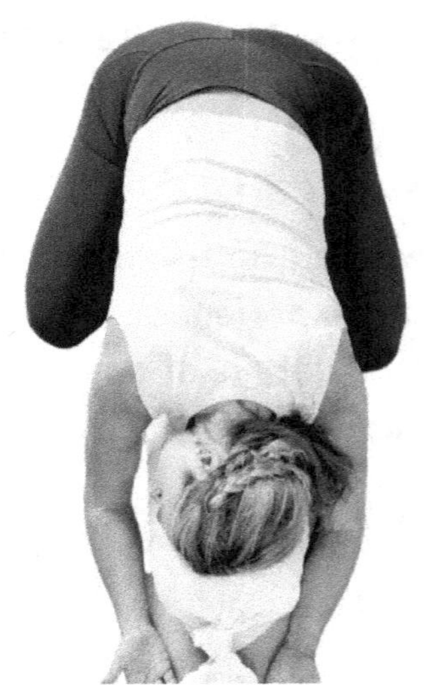

A Calming Method to Relieve Anxiety, Recharge, and Achieve Balance

Amy Orwell

Table of Contents

INTRODUCTION   **4**

Chapter 1:
History of Restorative Yoga   **6**

Chapter 2:
Benefits of Restorative Yoga   **11**

Chapter 3:
Tips for a Safe Restorative Yoga Practice   **17**

Chapter 4:
Props needed for Restorative Yoga   **20**

Chapter 5:
Visualization and Breathing in Restorative Yoga   **35**

Chapter 6:
Restorative Yoga Poses

    41

Chapter 7:
Assessing Your Progress   **77**

INTRODUCTION

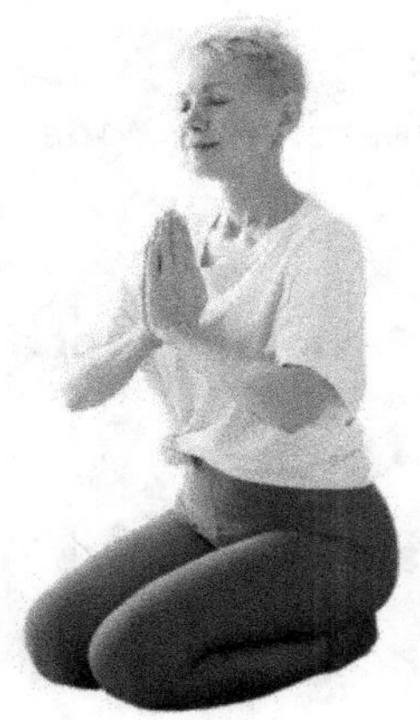

When I initially started doing yoga, I was going through the painful experience of losing my teenage daughter, I was looking for a way to de-stress, re-energize, and find my balance.

My acupuncturist encouraged me to try yoga, which I did and I have never looked back on it all these years because it relieved me from my grief and helped me find some peace.

In the same manner that yoga has been taught for many years, my instructors have passed on to me the information that is given in this book. Why then do I write this book? Why did I decide to impart my restorative yoga expertise to you? I will say it feels like the right time.

I have worked with countless individuals over the years, and one thing I wished for, was to find an easy and respected way to show and share knowledge on restorative yoga, and what better way than a book?

This book can be beneficial to you whether you're new to yoga, a seasoned practitioner, or have never tried it before. It will explain the philosophy of yoga and especially introduce you to restorative yoga if you have little to no familiarity with it.

The book will give readers with some background in yoga a clearer understanding of restorative yoga and how it differs from traditional yoga.

Chapter 1: History of Restorative Yoga

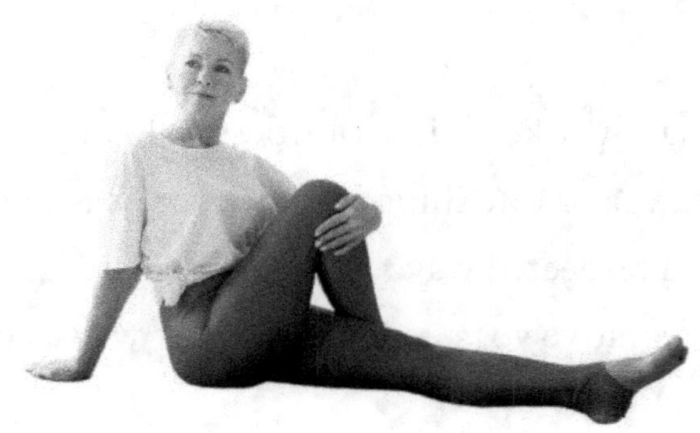

Yoga has a more than 5,000-year history in ancient Indian philosophy, and it is much more popular now. Individuals practice the activity for a variety of reasons, such as boosting flexibility, improving posture, strengthening their muscles, and overall wellness.

Before I give you detailed information on the history of restorative yoga, it is important you understand what restorative yoga means.

What is Restorative Yoga

A very soothing form of yoga practice is restorative yoga. It is not an active practice, but a passive one. Restorative yoga positions are maintained for five to twenty minutes, as opposed to the more vigorous forms of yoga when postures "flow" into one another.

With slow, soft movements or prolonged silence, restorative yoga aligns your physical and mental states. It also incorporates the idea of mindfulness, which enables practitioners to remain awake and aware of everything going on around them.

Restorative yoga is not only safe for older folks, but it also supports their physical and mental well-being. This form of yoga does not emphasize stretching or strengthening as traditional yoga does. In contrast to a typical yoga session, the asanas in this style are held for a longer period of time.

Yoga practitioners utilize props to deepen their practice and reach a state of total release and relaxation during a restorative yoga session. You may develop your self-soothing skills while learning the art of relaxation with restorative yoga. By nervous system rebalancing and stress response control, it can help seniors the ability to recover.

How did Restorative Yoga Begin

It's critical for you to understand the history of restorative yoga now that you are familiar with the term.

B.K.S. Iyengar, a yoga instructor, was a pioneer in the early 20th century in introducing the use of supports to assist those with physical limitations in doing asanas. Restorative yoga was not developed until the 1960s, but his lessons would eventually serve as inspiration for its creation.

Tirumalai Krishnamacharya, Iyengar's yoga instructor, and brother-in-law taught him the practice. Iyengar was a frail adolescent who used yoga to rebuild his strength.

He quickly rose to the status of a model student, even taking the place of one of Krishnamacharya's pupils in a yoga contest. Yoga tournaments were often held back then to display to the public the talent of these students.

Judith Hanson Lasater, an Iyengar student, began experimenting with employing props in ways that allowed participants to totally relax in the postures. She discovered that by maintaining the postures for extended lengths of time and using props like blankets, bolsters, and blocks for support, students were able to let go of stress and enter a profound state of relaxation.

In the 1970s, Lasater started teaching this form of yoga under the name "restorative yoga," and it immediately became well-liked. Other yoga instructors and practitioners started to create their own restorative yoga subcultures over time, each with its own methodology.

Chapter 2: Benefits of Restorative Yoga

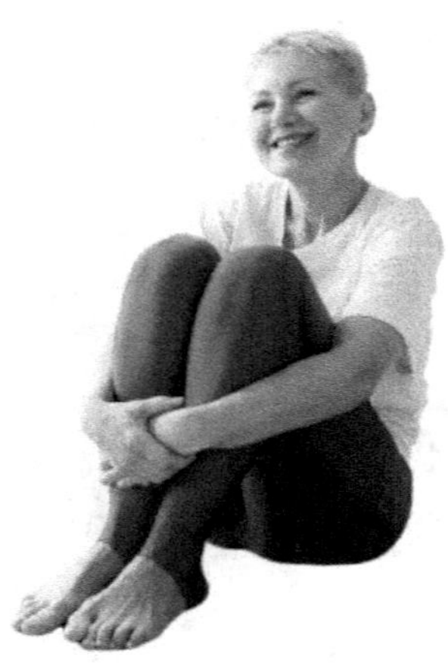

More than 14 million persons in the US who are over 50 practice yoga. The majority of older citizens include yoga in their everyday routines as a form of exercise. Some people do it as a part of their daily medical routine.

Seniors' flexibility, strength, and functional ability may all be improved by yoga in a secure manner. Seniors can benefit greatly from yoga, according to the National Recreation & Park Association. Besides the physical benefits, it gives elderly folks various other advantages.

I am aware of the case of Mr. Purushotaman, a 77-year-old man who had Parkinson's disease for four years. He participated in individualized yoga therapy, but for a long period, he observed little progress.

He continued to practice anyhow. After a few months, he noticed that his energy levels were increasing, especially when he was consistent throughout his asana and pranayama routine.

This exercise can aid in your recovery if you've had stress, trauma, accident, or sickness. This practice will assist you in maintaining your physical well-being if you are a regular person with typical levels of stress in your life.

Self-discovery can be facilitated through restorative yoga. By bringing the mind's awareness of the limitations of the body, it aids in developing harmony between the mind and body. You get a better knowledge of your emotional state and may pinpoint the underlying reasons for any discomfort or suffering as you become more in tune with your physical self. The benefits include:

Now we proceed to discuss the actual benefits of restorative yoga for you as a senior:

Helps you recover following a surgical procedure: Restorative yoga promotes relaxation, so when you practice it, you'll have more energy, which will aid in your healing. You may also speed up your recovery from particular surgeries by adopting particular positions and movements.

Decreases Obesity: Restorative yoga can be a surprise solution to enabling overweight men and women still lose weight when high-intensity aerobic activity—which is shown to burn calories and decrease fat—is just not practicable. Restorative yoga lowers the amount of cortisol in your body, according to studies.

According to research, doing restorative yoga instead of a more rigorous type will help you burn weight more effectively. Reduced cortisol synthesis also results in a reduction in the body's capacity to produce glucose. Glucose causes fat to be produced, particularly belly fat, which can also result in other illnesses.

Enhances Respiration: As people age, they encounter a variety of respiratory issues that can be harmful to their health. Because of this, the body receives less oxygen, which can be harmful to your general health. According to research, an adult yoga practice lasting three months can help senior women breathe better. A fundamental aspect of life is breathing. Even though you may go days without eating, you cannot go even a few minutes without breathing, thus as you age, it is important to maintain a healthy respiratory system.

Lowers high blood pressure: The most common ailment affecting the elderly nowadays is hypertension. Several clinical trials have demonstrated that older people's oxidative stress is reduced by yoga treatment. One of the main causes of hypertension in the elderly is oxidative stress.

Anxiety is Reduced by Restorative Yoga: Yoga programs, especially restorative yoga for older persons, aid in mental and physical relaxation. It helps ease tension and anxiety in elderly folks when frequently performed. This is because it emphasizes slow, deep breathing and motions to stimulate the neural system.

Alleviates the discomfort of menopause: Menopausal swings can be stressful, but some yoga positions might help you manage it. To relieve menopausal symptoms, you might practice positions like the Bridge.

Strengthens Your Bones: Weight-bearing workouts like yoga are believed to help prevent bone density loss and lower osteoporosis. Yoga activities can be helpful if you're trying to treat or prevent osteoporosis or reduce pain following a bone fracture.

More Flexibility: Restorative yoga is a better choice if you're looking for gentle stretches that will increase your flexibility. If you have tight or sore joints, flexibility exercises like restorative yoga are excellent. Researchers recently determined that restorative yoga provides therapeutic advantages after looking at how well yoga therapy managed arthritis in elderly women.

Blood Circulation is Enhanced: Your hands and feet's circulation can be improved with the yoga relaxation techniques you learn. This guarantees that your cells receive enough amount of oxygen, which helps your body work properly.

Alleviates sciatica: Pain that originates in the buttocks and travels down the leg occurs when the sciatic nerve is stimulated and becomes inflamed. Several positions used in restorative yoga induce traction, which relieves strain on the nerve.

Chapter 3: Tips for a Safe Restorative Yoga Practice

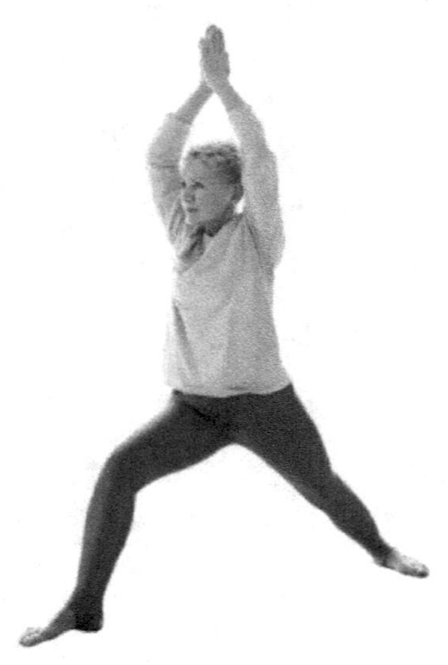

Seniors should be able to practice yoga safely. Even though yoga is supposed to be simple, if a posture is new, difficult, or unfamiliar, it's possible to hurt yourself.

Yoga that is soft and calming, such as restorative yoga, tries to soothe the mind, lessen tension, and encourage physical relaxation. Yet, it is crucial to exercise carefully to prevent harm and treat existing medical concerns.

Here are some tips for safe restorative yoga practice:

<u>This is not a contest</u>- Remember that yoga is not a sport that requires competition. Never evaluate yourself against other yogis or yoginis. Concentrate on a few positions at a time while moving at your own pace.

<u>The muscles should be warmed up</u> - Warming up the muscles before doing yoga is advised. Without a proper warm-up, assuming a full stance can strain your muscles.

<u>If required, use props</u>- Everyone is unique. Some people are unable to fully extend out when performing certain asanas. Learn to use props in this situation, like chairs, blocks, pillows, bolsters, and whatever else works for you.

<u>Practice within your limitations -</u> The goal of restorative yoga is not to achieve extreme flexibility or to push oneself to the limit. Keep your movements light and within your comfort range.

<u>The form is secondary to function -</u> People frequently want to do a certain asana flawlessly on their first attempt. At starting, it is less important how the stance seems. The muscles and bone structure of seniors are already feeble. Encouragement of safe yoga practices is therefore essential. Find the difference between challenging yourself and straining even as you do so.

Chapter 4: Props needed for Restorative Yoga

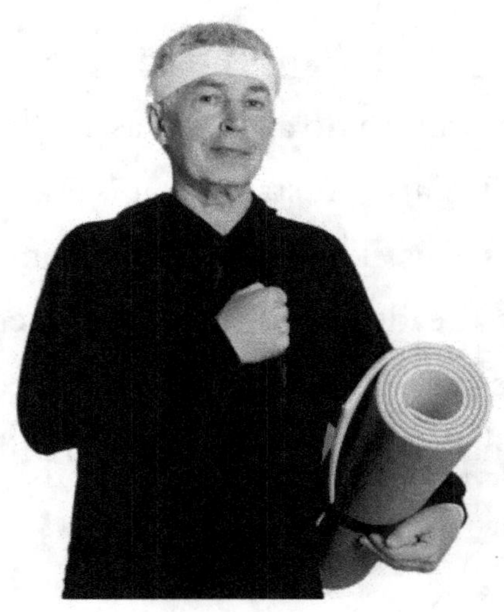

Male ascetics who gave up material belongings and led solitary lives in search of enlightenment were the main teachers and practitioners of yoga.

Yet a few trailblazing female practitioners who went against the accepted gender roles in the early 20th century brought yoga to the West. These women, such as Indra Devi, Tara Michael, and Lilias Folan, introduced yoga to the West and opened it up to women of various ages and socioeconomic backgrounds.

At the time, many people had doubts about yoga's advantages for women since they believed it to be largely a male discipline. Yet, these women persisted and contributed to the acceptance of yoga as a form of exercise and stress alleviation for women, opening the door for the development of the current yoga business that we are familiar with today.

What precisely do you need to practice restorative yoga now that you are aware of what it is and how it might assist you in achieving physical and mental balance?

You will learn what you need and how to use the many props that restorative yoga uses to help you feel supported and comfortable in this chapter.

Also, you should make sure that you have a physical area where you feel safe and at ease in which to practice. Also, you'll learn how to set up your area for restorative yoga.

After all, it's challenging to relax and extend your body if you are concerned that someone is about to intrude or that your tranquility is being disturbed by a cell phone that keeps ringing. Let's look at everything you need to prepare for restorative yoga.

Organizing the Space

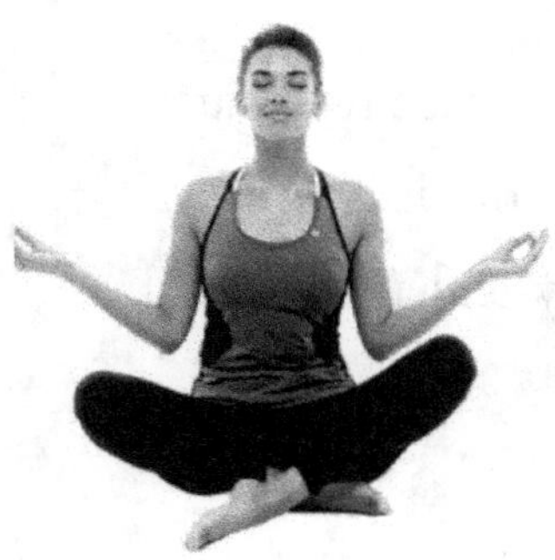

Consider one word: comfort, while preparing a setting for your restorative yoga practice. You'll need to design an environment that will enable you to unwind completely. These are some essential ideas to keep in mind when arranging the area:

- <u>Get your watch off -</u> If you want to fully let go, avoid wearing a watch while you practice since it symbolizes your ties to time. To measure how long you spend in each posture, use a timer with a melodic chime as an alternative.

- <u>Warm room temperature -</u> Warmth should permeate the space, and you should dress accordingly. Keep additional layers on hand. Being chilly prevents relaxation. It's a good idea to prepare in advance since when you rest, your internal temperature will drop.

- <u>Reduce noise -</u> Make sure there is as little outside noise as possible in your location. Relaxing music is good, but even the most calming music might occasionally prevent you from genuinely being able to let go because of the ideas that arise while you listen. Ensure that nothing may distract you while you work.

- <u>Dark Space -</u> While strong light will keep you overstimulated, start by making sure the area you're in is as dark as possible.

Blocks

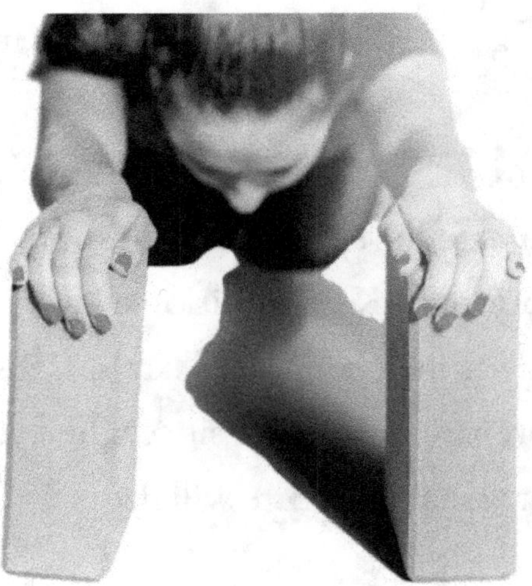

Before beginning restorative yoga, make sure you have at least two blocks available. Blocks can be produced from foam, wood, or cork. I advise choosing some constructed firm foam.

Thick foam blocks are stronger than the other types and softer than cork or wood when put directly on the body. Blocks are useful since they may support weak points in your body, are really simple to use, and don't take up much room. I advise choosing blocks that are 4", 6", and 9" in size. (Short, medium, and tall are the three conventional heights for each block.)

Bolsters

In restorative yoga, the main prop you use to support yourself while in a position is a bolster. In an ideal world, you would have a flat and a circular bolster for your practice, but if necessary, you can make bolsters out of blankets. About 8" 27" 32.5" for flat bolsters and 9" 26" 34.5 for circular bolsters.

 These dimensions are significant if you plan to replicate them using blankets. All of the postures and sequences may be done with one of these two bolsters. When you practice, use whatever feels natural to you.

Blankets

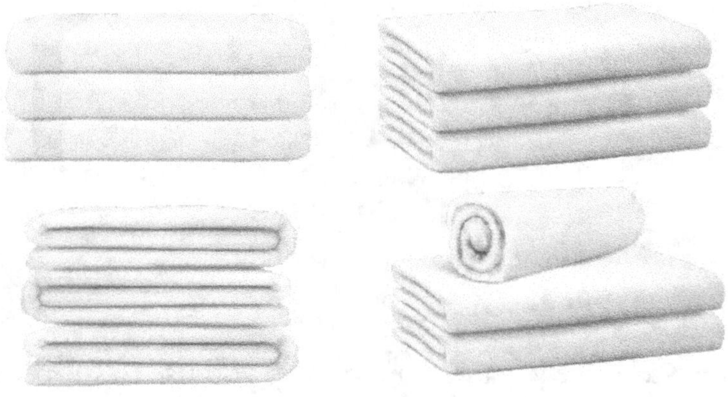

During restorative yoga sessions, blankets offer additional warmth and comfort. Wool or Mexican-style blankets composed of cotton or a cotton/wool combination are the two most common materials used in traditional yoga blankets.

 If utilizing a blanket from your house, bear in mind that you should use one that is around 75" x 52".

You'll feel more at ease in the positions thanks to the weight of the blanket. Another option is to swaddle yourself in a blanket, which will subtly remind you of how it feels to be a newborn being cared for, instantly calming you down. Moreover, blankets may be piled to make a bolster, or they can be utilized to offer complete or partial support.

You should be aware of all the many ways a blanket can be used and handled since there are so many different ways you may utilize it. Some of the important folds are listed here, including Half fold, open fold, oblong fold, square fold, small square, short and long roll, accordion, headrest fold, and rectangle fold.

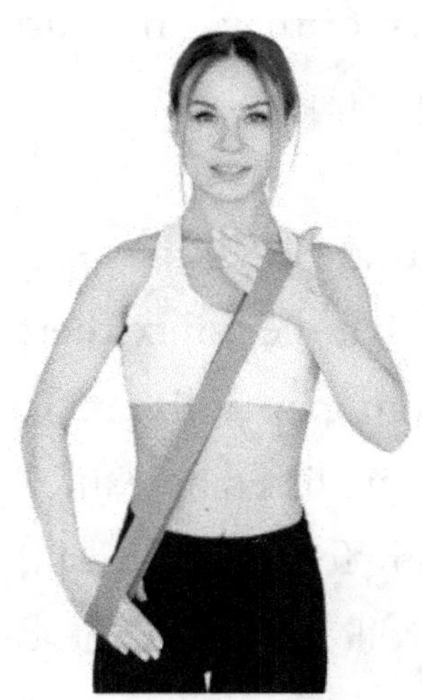

In order to extend your body, straps are frequently utilized in yoga. For instance, the strap allows you to reach your feet even if you can't with your hands. In order to acquire a suitable stretch, you may also utilize them as a tool.

They are employed in restorative yoga as a means of establishing stability. A strap is a crucial restorative yoga prop because it offers support while allowing you to relax into a stretch without exertion.

Most choices are provided with a 10-inch strap belt. Because they provide the quickest means of entering and exiting, quick-release belts are my favorite. But if you don't have the opportunity to buy a suitable yoga strap, you may use any sort you have or even an old tie.

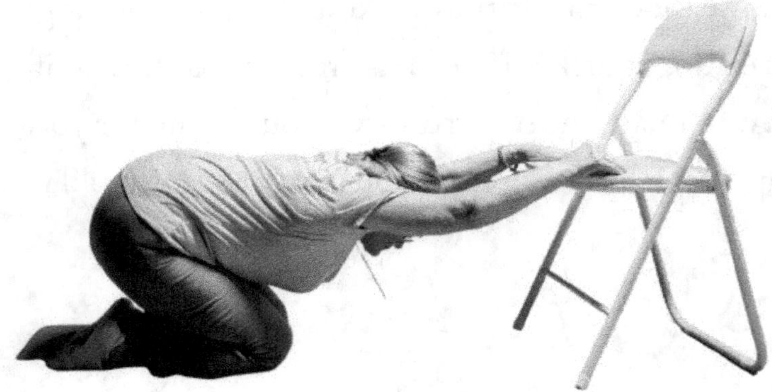

The ideal chair to utilize has a flat seat, such as those found in conventional folding chairs or special yoga chairs without backs. Several yoga supply stores have backless chairs, which are a little simpler to use than standard folding chairs.

When using a folding chair, ensure sure it is well-built. Insufficient support in your chair makes it difficult to unwind. An alternative to a bolster or a wall in some situations is a chair.

Sandbags

In restorative yoga, sandbags are used for "grounding," which is placing them on particular body regions to impart weight to those areas. The practice of grounding is crucial because it enhances the sense of security that promotes relaxation and promotes healing. If you don't want to spend the money on sandbags explicitly made for yoga, a ten-pound bag of rice covered in a pillowcase will do.

Eye Bag/ Eye Pillows

Every restorative yoga position would benefit from the inclusion of eye bags or cushions since they can assist to relax the eyes and block out light. Keep them close at reach to intensify the calm you experience

Headwrap

The traditional headband used in yoga resembles an ACE bandage. It is firmly wrapped around the head to exert a soothing pressure that promotes relaxation. Yet, they are excellent to use at any time. Headwraps are mostly utilized in poses that address migraines and heat stress.

Yoga Mat

A yoga mat is helpful for any position that requires you to sit or lie down. If you're training on one, it offers additional protection from the hard floor. A yoga mat can save you from slipping when performing standing poses or more challenging ones that include chairs. Yoga mats also give you a tidy area in which to practice. You can use a big towel or blanket in its place if you don't have a yoga mat.

Wall

This book contains a number of postures that call for a wall since restorative yoga uses it as a primary source of support. The good news is that you can find walls wherever you go without having to buy them. To practice restorative yoga in your home, you might wish to clear a wall area. When you return to that wall, you will feel truly "at home" since you will utilize it repeatedly.

Employ What Works

Several positions may be put up with only a few props, and you might even be able to utilize items you already have at home to practice without spending a fortune on new equipment. For instance, pillows and couch cushions make excellent bolsters, while a necktie serves as a useful yoga strap.

You may use books as "blocks," a washcloth as an "eye cushion," and additional household blankets and towels as "blankets." You shouldn't feel pressured to buy every yoga accessory available on the market. But don't cut corners: The more the merrier when it comes to props! Always feel free to include more props as necessary. There is simply never enough. Comfort is key, and when you're at ease, you can heal well.

Chapter 5: Visualization and Breathing in Restorative Yoga

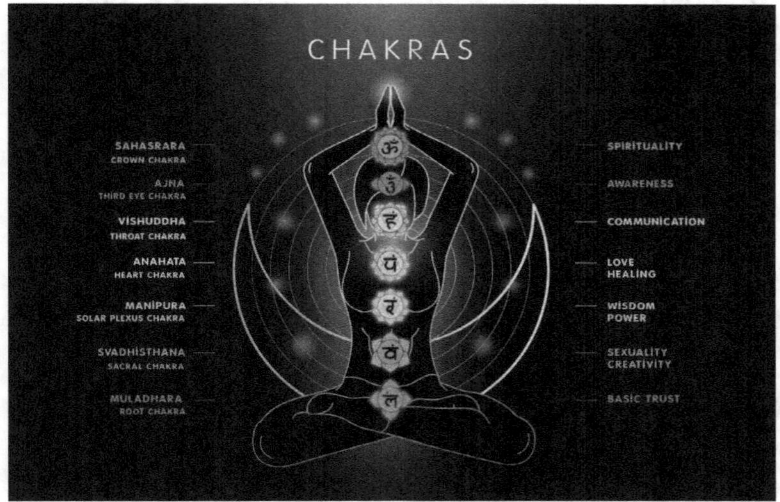

The chakras and the breath are said to be closely related in yoga and other ancient Indian systems like Ayurveda and Tantra. Along the body's central axis are energy centers known as chakras. Each chakra is connected to certain attributes, activities, and elements, such as the breath.

The chakras may be balanced and activated by using different pranayama or breathing methods, which can also assist to control and harmonize the breath. This promotes physical, emotional, and spiritual well-being. These are some instances of how the chakras and respiration are related:

Root Chakra (Muladhara): The root chakra is related to the element of earth and is linked with stability and grounding. While doing root chakra pranayama, it might be beneficial to concentrate on the exhale, which aids in letting go of extra energy and stress in the body and to picture the breath descending into the ground.

Sacral Chakra (Svadhisthana): The sacral chakra is related to the element of water and is tied to creativity and sexuality. It might be beneficial to concentrate on the inhale, which aids in nourishing and replenishing the body and to picture the breath moving down the lower abdomen like a wave while doing pranayama for the sacral chakra.

<u>Solar Plexus Chakra (Manipura):</u> The solar plexus chakra is linked to the element of fire and is related to one's own strength and willpower. It might be beneficial to concentrate on the breath of fire, a quick and vigorous breath that aids in activating and energizing the body while doing pranayama for the solar plexus chakra.

<u>Heart Chakra (Anahata):</u> The element of air is linked to the heart chakra, which is related to feelings of love and compassion. Focusing on the breath of love, a slow, deep breath that aids in opening and expanding the heart center, might be beneficial while doing pranayama for the heart chakra.

<u>Throat Chakra (Vishuddha):</u> The throat chakra is linked to the element of ether or space and is related to self-expression and communication. It might be beneficial to concentrate on the ujjayi breath, a deep and loud breath that aids in cleansing and clearing the throat and airways while doing pranayama for the throat chakra.

Third Eye Chakra (Ajna): The third eye chakra is linked to the element of light and is tied to intuition and spiritual understanding. Focusing on the shambhavi mudra, a gaze or vision that helps to concentrate and guide the energy of the breath onto the third eye may be beneficial while doing pranayama for the third eye chakra.

Crown Chakra (Sahasrara): The element of awareness is tied to the crown chakra, which is connected to transcendence and spiritual enlightenment. Focusing on the Sahaj or spontaneous breath, a natural and easy breath that aids in unifying and harmonizing the body, mind, and spirit, may be beneficial while doing pranayama for the crown chakra.

Relaxation, stress alleviation, and restoring the body's natural equilibrium are the main goals of the gentle and therapeutic yoga style known as restorative yoga. A crucial component of this practice, breathing, and visualization exercises aid in stress relief, and mental calmness, and increase the practice's overall health benefits.

The most popular breathing and visualization techniques used in restorative yoga include the following:

Diaphragmatic Breathing: This method, sometimes referred to as belly breathing, is inhaling through the nose while letting the abdomen expand. Release all of the air from your tummy by exhaling through your mouth. Repeat a few times, paying attention to your breathing and letting your body relax.

Alternate Nostril Breathing: This method is breathing in through one nostril while covering the other with the thumb, and then exhaling while covering the first nostril with the ring finger. Repeat a few times, paying attention to your breathing and unwinding your body.

<u>Box Breathing:</u> This method is breathing for four counts, holding the breath for four counts, expelling for four counts, and then holding the breath for four counts. Repeat a few times, paying attention to your breathing and unwinding your body.

Chapter 6: Restorative Yoga Poses

It's time to look at the different restorative yoga poses that will enable you to find comfort in your body, recover from illness or physical injury, and gain a sense of balance and well-being now that you are aware of Chakras and are familiar with the breathing techniques that will help you get ready for restorative yoga.

Remember that there is no one right method to choose the restorative yoga postures from this chapter.

You may practice one position at a time or mix and combine according on what seems natural to your body that day. You can find that a certain stance makes you feel something physically or emotionally.

Pay close attention to such emotions. Consider their possible sources of origin. It is advantageous to practice with this degree of awareness since it will enable your practice to come more intuitively. In the end, if you pay attention, you already possess the knowledge to cure yourself.

The more you do these postures, the more you'll discover which ones speak to you and aid in reestablishing some balance in the areas of your body that most need it.

While you attempt these postures, keep in mind that every person's physique is unique and that certain poses will suit you better than others.

For instance, depending on your degree of flexibility and fitness, certain positions may be particularly difficult to enter.

Allow yourself the opportunity to explore, and don't hurry, as you spend some time determining what suits you with each stance. Keep in mind that you need to feel secure and at ease in order to unwind completely.

Now let us start exploring these poses and help you find your way to better health.

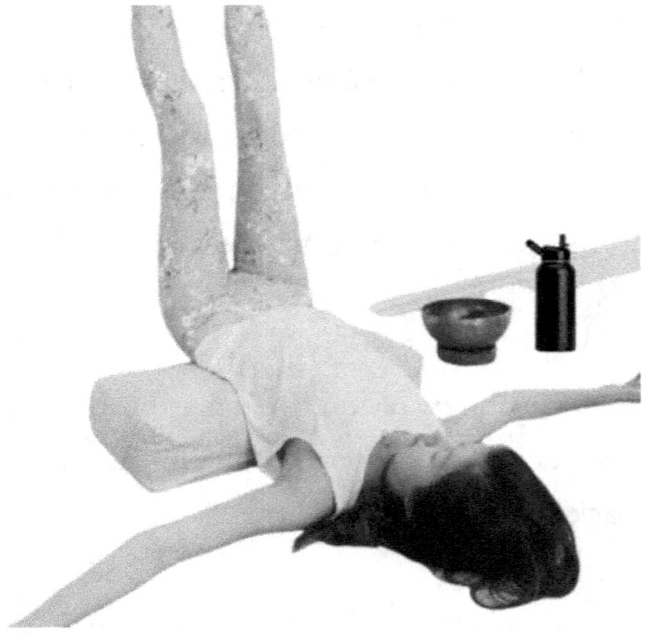

Many people love this posture because it has many of the same health advantages as a back bend and is a fantastic overall restorative position.

It revitalizes worn-out legs and feet, relaxes the nervous system, and is excellent for restoring your energy when traveling since it promotes blood circulation after extended periods of sitting. Even your legs' swelling, a typical problem brought on by flying, is reduced by it.

The posture is not too difficult to do. The advantage of the position is claimed to have the same impact on your nervous system as taking a sleep for 20 minutes (but an awake nap—stay connected to your breath!), as the stance has the same effect on your nervous system.

Because of how restorative it may be, the position provides many of the same physical advantages as a back bend.

Since it might be risky to lie flat on your back during the second and third trimesters of pregnancy, this position is not advised.

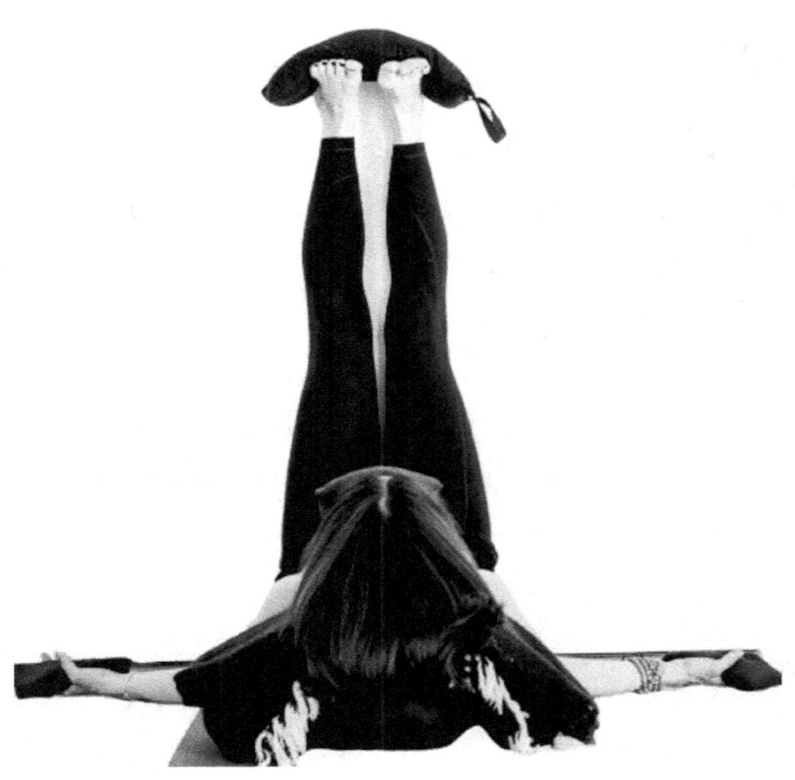

Props needed:

Mat

Sandbag

Blanket (Head Rest Fold) (optional)

Bolster

Strap

The Process:

- The long side of a bolster should be placed against the block after a block of the same height as the long side against the wall has been placed.

- If desired, place a Rectangular Fold blanket on top of the center of the bolster and wrap it over it to create a T-shape. The remaining blanket should be placed on your mat.

- Place one hip on the bolster as you sit sideways, then drop your shoulder and head to the floor next to you.

- Stretch your legs up the wall as you roll onto your back, then adjust your posture such that your tailbone is tilted up over the bolster.

- Spread your arms out in a T- or U-shape to the sides. Roll up the Rectangular Fold blanket that is in the center of your mat to support your neck if required.

- Get comfortable and focus on your breathing. A minimum of five and a maximum of twenty minutes should be spent maintaining this position.

- Bend your knees, move the bolster closer to the wall to exit the position, and then roll to your right side to stand up.

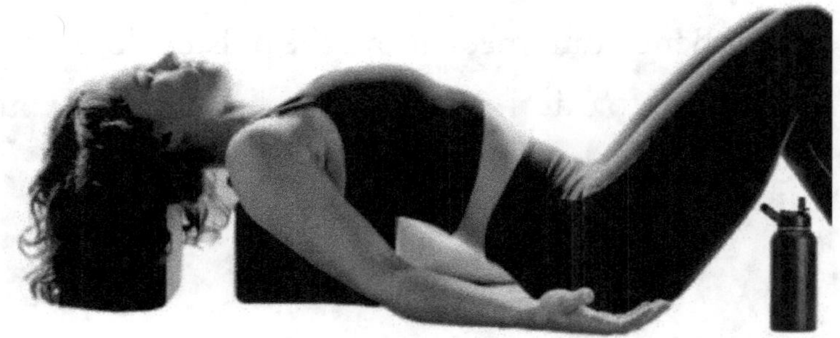

The immune system is controlled by the thymus gland, which is situated in the middle of the chest behind the upper breastbone.

If the thymus gland is stimulated, the immune system will also be. Open-chest poses, like the Fish Pose, aid in strengthening your immune system so it can more effectively combat foreign invaders like germs and viruses. But Fish Pose may also relax the immune system when practiced in restorative yoga, which is especially beneficial during allergy season when the immune system is working overtime.

This position expands the neck as well if you practice it with only one block beneath your back. To gain the best from Fish Pose, take a deep breath into the chest. With or without a bolster placed on top of the blocks, this stance may be performed.

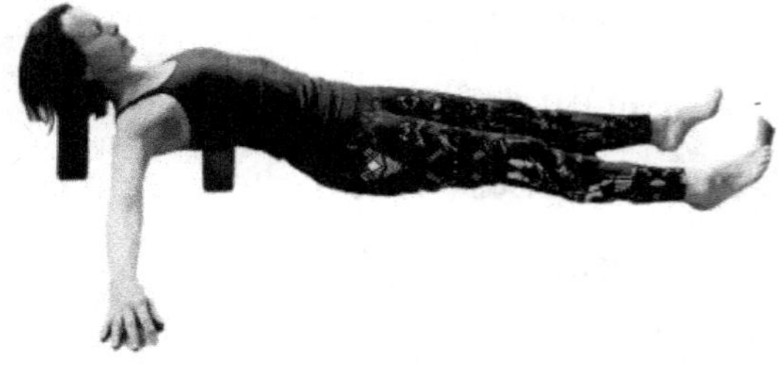

Props needed:

Mat

2 blocks

Headwrap (optional)

1-2 bolsters (optional)

The Process:

- If you're using blocks, spread them out on your mat two at a time. The pair may be made up of either a short and tall block or a medium and short block. If you're using a bolster, place one over each set of blocks or place it flat on the floor.

- Legs extended in front of you, lie back over the blocks or bolster. Spend at least five minutes concentrating on your breathing and expanding your chest. If it makes you more comfortable and relaxed, feel free to wear a headwrap. You may bend your legs if you want, and put a second bolster below them for support. Your palms should be facing up or toward your body when you rest your arms by your side.

- To exit, roll to your side and budge your knees. Roll back onto your back while maintaining a bent knee position. Push the blocks and/or bolsters out of the way. Consider how much more open your chest region feels now. After you've adjusted, roll to your side and rise to a sitting position.

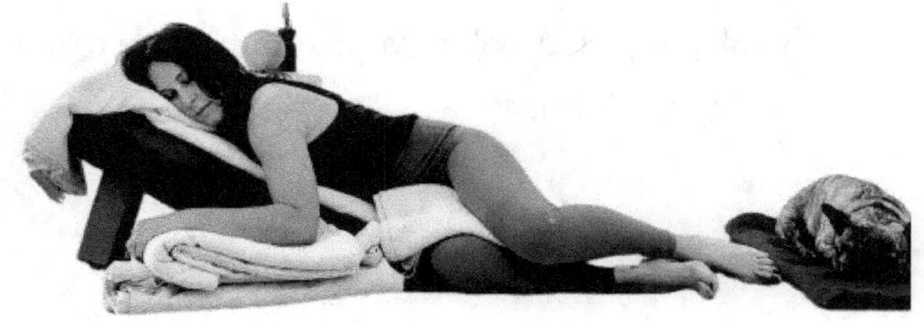

This position is a calming variation where you may experience complete relaxation. It calms your breathing and eases stress and tension in the muscles that run down the sides and in the middle of your torso, which adds to a general sense of calm.

Don't be afraid; this mild stance is really suitable for everybody, even those who have back issues or are pregnant.

Props needed:
Mat
Bolster
2-4 blankets (rectangle fold)
2 blocks

The Process:

- The center of the mat should have the bolster placed lengthwise. Your blankets and blocks should be close by.

- While you sit in front of the bolster, raise your right hip up to it while bending your knees, letting them fall into a comfortable position.

- Make sure you feel cozy and supported by experimenting with the bolster. You may opt to use blocks to elevate the bolster at an angle (use a short and medium pair or a medium and tall pair), or you can lay a Rectangular Fold blanket over the bolster to provide support for your head.

- Lower your bottom arm to the floor next to the bolster and then extend it along it. Your upper hand should be on the bolster's opposite side. Lower yourself to the bolster by angling your tummy in its direction. Inhale as you move, stretch your spine, then breathe out and twist a bit more. You may either turn your head towards the direction of your knees or, for a deeper twist, away from them. If you did not turn away from your knees at first, you could discover that when your body begins to relax after a few minutes, you can turn your head to the side of the deeper twist. Let the bolster be your support: Try not to hold yourself up by relaxing your arms. To relieve any back strain you may be experiencing, if necessary, insert a blanket or block between your knees. For further comfort, you may raise your arms on two blankets in the shape of a rectangle at an angle so that your hands are higher than your elbows.

- Maintain this stance for three minutes, then release it by pushing off the bolster while sitting up with your hands on the floor. Repeat to the left.

Child's Pose

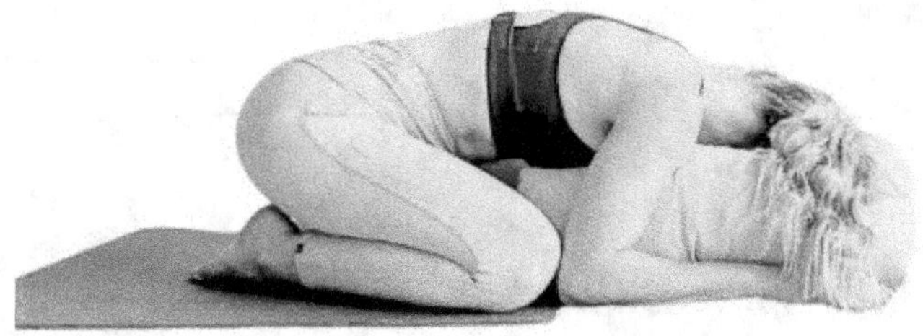

The fundamental yoga posture for relaxation is the child's pose. It's a "safe" posture where you may engage with your breath and feel loved and supported.

Child's Pose is a fantastic forward bend that works to softly loosen up the back of the body and massage the abdominal organs on a physical level. It's crucial that you don't feel like you're supporting yourself in this position; instead, let the bolster or chairs do the supporting so that you may relax completely.

Props needed:

Mat

1-2 bolster

Blankets (optional)

2 blocks (optional)

The Process:

- Put a half-folded (lengthwise) blanket on the floor if you feel like your knees could use some additional cushioning. Have a Square Fold blanket close hand to place below your feet if your feet are narrow. As much as you need for comfort, roll the blanket up.

- Sit back to rest on your heels while holding the bolster's narrow end between your knees. Your whole tummy should be on the bolster as you lean forward. By angling the bolster and using two blocks of varying heights—short and medium or medium and tall—you may lift it higher. The blocks should support the bolster's midsection and head. To provide extra support for the low back, if needed, insert a Long Roll Fold blanket at the crease of your hip and thigh.

- Put a Rectangle Fold blanket under each arm if it is uncomfortable for them to lay on the floor or if they don't reach it. To create a comfortable place for your hands to rest, you may fold the top of the blanket beneath.

- After a short while, move your head to one side before doing the opposite. Give each side the same amount of time.

- At least five minutes should be spent in the position. Move the bolster to the side and gradually uncurl your body once you're done. You should also extend your legs.

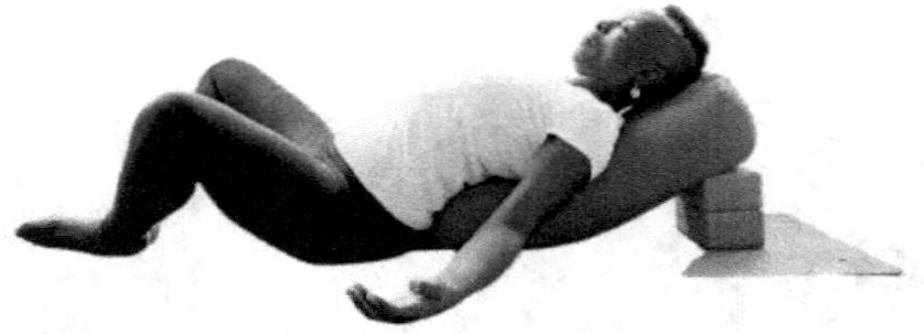

In restorative yoga, this position is a favorite. When it extends your inner thighs, opens up your pelvic region, and opens up your back and hips, it promotes relaxation.

Supta Baddha Konasana, also known as Supported Bound Angle Pose, is a restorative yoga position that gently stretches the hips and inner thighs. This position is perfect for anyone who spends a lot of time sitting, has lower back problems, or needs to de-stress and unwind.

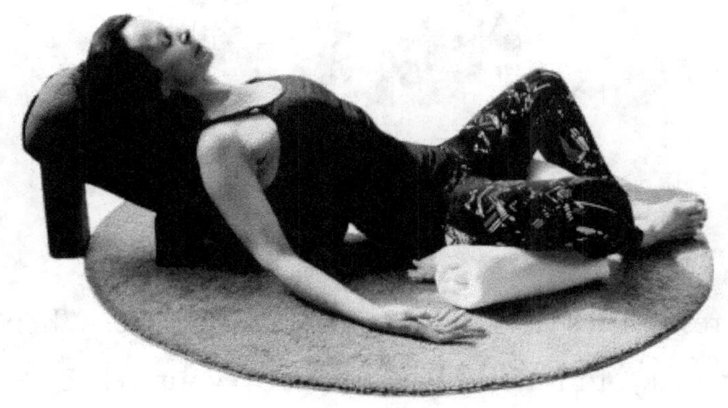

Props needed:

Mat

Bolster

2 blocks

2 blankets

The Process:

- Two blocks should be spaced closely apart on your mat. The pair may be made up of either a short and tall block or a medium and short block. Suspend a bolster from the blocks.

- Bring your lower back all the way up to the bolster's lowest narrow end while sitting on the floor.

- With your chest pulled forward and your back slightly bent, place your hands on the bolster behind you and recline over it.

- Your knees should hang out to the sides as you bring your foot soles together.

- Placing the blanket in the Head Rest Fold under your head can provide additional support if needed for your neck. Use two blankets folded in the short roll as tiny bolsters beneath your knees if you feel like your legs might need extra support. Instead, you may

cover your whole body with the Open Fold
blanket. Your palms should be facing up as you
rest your hands on your thighs or let your arms
hang down next to you.

- By putting your hands on the outside of your
  thighs, you may draw your legs together to exit
  this position. After a brief period of
  adjustment, roll to your right side and rise to a
  sitting position.

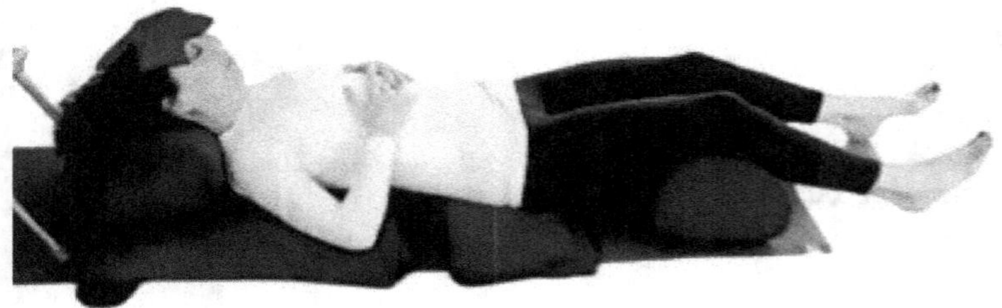

In restorative yoga, heart-opening postures are intended to reduce upper-back and chest tension while simultaneously encouraging sentiments of openness, compassion, and love.

These positions are particularly advantageous for those who spend a lot of time sitting, slouching over a computer, or who are feeling pressured or nervous.

Props needed:
2-3 bolster
Mat
Blankets

The Process:

- Put a bolster beneath your shoulder blades and midback on one side of the mat, and place another bolster under your knees on the other.

- Spread your arms out in a T-shape over the top of the bolsters under your shoulders as you lay over them. You may replace the first bolster with a Rectangle Fold blanket beneath your shoulders if it seems too high, or you can lay a Head Rest Fold blanket under your head.

- Maintain this posture for no less than five minutes or more than twenty minutes. Pay close attention to how deeply and thoroughly you're breathing in.

- Place your feet on the bolster that is under your knees and push them away to exit the posture. Roll to your right side while bending your knees. The top bolster may now be moved toward your head if you'd want to use it as a cushion at this stage. You should give yourself some time to acclimate before standing up to the seat.

<u>**Reclining Hero Pose**</u>

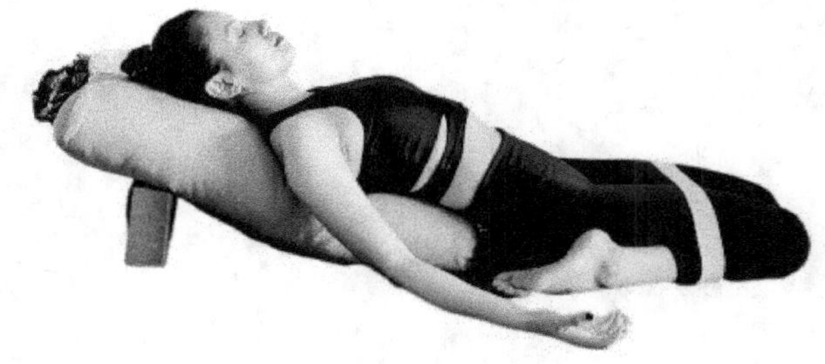

rigid back? You may be shocked to hear that tight quadriceps might be to blame! A great way to relieve lower back strain is to do the reclining hero pose, which stretches the quadriceps, abdomen, and deep hip flexor. This position aids digestion and respiration in addition to being helpful for back problems.

While it will be difficult if you have tight quadriceps or knee problems, it gets simpler with the support used in restorative yoga. Depending on your requirements, you may alter this stance. Keep the posture for each variation for at least five minutes.

Props needed:

Mat

Bolster

2 blankets (optional)

2-4 blocks

The Process:

- Kneel in front of the bolster, position a block at a short or medium height there to support your buttocks, and then place another block (at a height that feels good) beneath the head end of the bolster to angle it before you lay back on it. If the bolster has to be lifted higher, maintain the angle by placing a block at a medium or tall height under the head end and a short or medium height block under the end closest to your spine. You may use the blankets as armrests by placing one on either side of you in the Long Roll Fold.

- Put your hands on the floor and push up to sit up straight to exit this position on your hands and knees. Next, to get your legs' blood flowing again, extend each leg backward individually.

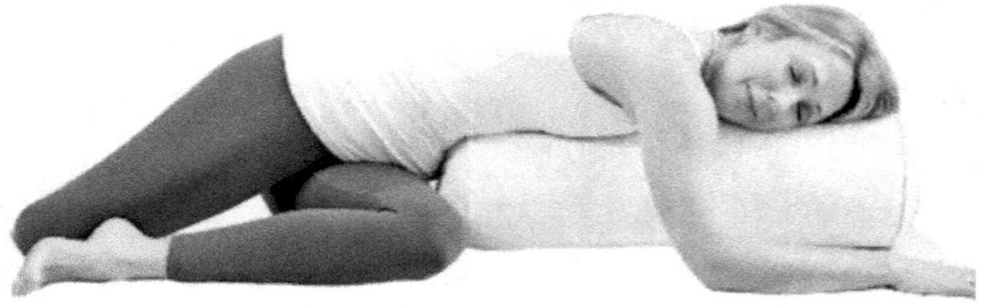

Due to the compression of the internal spaces, closed twists like this one tend to exert a deeper strain on the abdominal organs than open twists. Although restorative postures should be restful, this one offers a little bit more stretch on the side of your lower leg, and sometimes a little bit more stretch may eventually help your body relax more profoundly.

Everyone may do this position to some extent, but it is particularly beneficial for runners and cyclists since it helps to loosen the iliotibial band, a ligament that often aggravates during these sports.

Props needed:

Bolster

Mat

2 blocks (optional)

2-4 blankets (optional)

The Process:

- Your mat's midsection should have the bolster placed lengthwise. Blocks and blankets should be kept close by.

- With your knees bent, start sitting in front of the bolster and then raise your right hip to it.

- Your lower leg should now be fully extended and parallel to the bolster. Your upper leg should now be parallel to your body when you straighten it.

- Turn your belly toward the bolster while holding the sides of the bolster with both hands. If you want a deeper twist, tilt your head away from your upper leg as you squat down to the bolster. If you did not initially move away, you could discover that when your body begins to relax after a few minutes, you are able to turn your head to the side of the deeper twist.

- To ensure that your back is properly positioned and at ease when it rests on the bolster, experiment with it. Using blocks (use a short and medium pair or a medium and big pair), you may choose to lift the bolster at an angle. You can also opt to support your head by laying a Rectangular Fold blanket over the mat widthwise.

- Relax your arms and let the bolster support you; avoid using your arms as a means of

self-support. To ease any tension that doesn't
seem natural, you might opt to gently bend
your legs. At least three minutes should be
spent in this position.

- Pressing your hands into the floor will help you
release the stance. Afterward, sit up straight.
the left side, repeat

Revolved abdomen pose

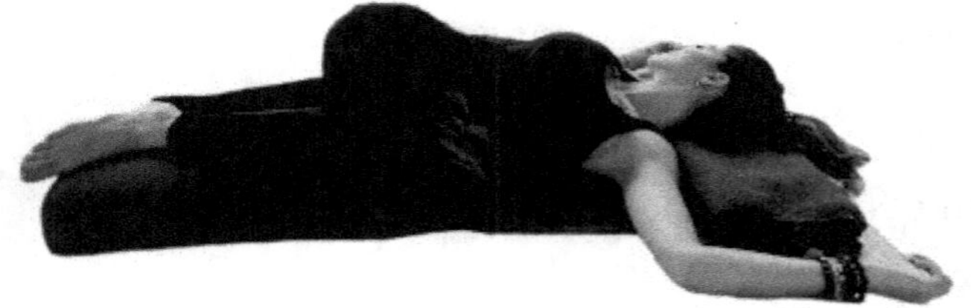

One of the most rewarding yoga positions is the revolving abdomen stance. Twisting causes your body to push against itself, which naturally releases tension without any effort. In this position, the lower back and abdominal muscles receive a good workout, which benefits the digestive system.

This twist is performed in restorative yoga while your hips are lifted on a bolster for additional support. Be open to releasing all the poisons from your center while you are in the position. (Use a blanket in the shape of a rectangle if the bolster is too high for your hips in this posture.)

Props needed:
2 bolsters
Mat
Blankets (optional)

The Process:

- The middle of your mat should have a bolster placed across it. By raising your legs up toward your chest and bending your knees, you may lay down on your left side with your bottom arm parallel to the bolster while sitting in the center of the bolster. Ensure that your right leg crosses completely over your torso and that your left knee rests with its back to the ground. As your left hip is positioned on the bolster, your right hip will be in the air. A second bolster should be placed between your legs. If your lower leg needs more support, place a blanket in a rectangular shape below it. It's important to keep in mind that you should twist from your torso, not your knees, as you attempt to make a 90-degree angle with your torso and legs across the floor.

- Your back, head, and arms should all rest on the floor while you recline with your arms outstretched in a T-shape. Always maintain the original position for your hips and legs. By putting a blanket in the Head Rest Fold beneath your head, you may support it if it's unpleasant. Maintain your right hand on your ribcage while relaxing your elbow toward the ground if your right shoulder is bothersome. Spend at least three minutes in this posture.

- Bring your right arm to your left side, sit up, and lift your head last to exit the posture. Pose again from the other side.

Chapter 7: Assessing Your Progress

Creating a sensation of relaxation and healing in the body and mind is the aim of restorative yoga.

It might be useful for seniors who practice restorative yoga to monitor their development over time to see whether they are reaping the benefits they anticipate from the practice. The following are some methods for seniors to gauge their success with restorative yoga:

Physical changes: Seeing physical changes in the body is one approach to gauging restorative yoga development. Seniors could see better posture, more flexibility, and less discomfort or stress in their bodies.

Mental changes: The practice of restorative yoga may be beneficial for mental health. Seniors who frequently practice restorative yoga may discover that it helps them feel more at ease, composed, and less anxious.

Improved sleep: Seniors who practice restorative yoga may also see changes in their sleeping habits. They could discover that they can sleep better and longer, which can improve their general health and well-being.

Consistency: Looking at how regularly one has been practicing restorative yoga is another approach to gauge development. Restorative yoga may be more beneficial for seniors who have been able to maintain a regular practice routine.

Ability to hold poses: Seniors may discover that they can hold restorative yoga positions for extended periods of time with practice. This could indicate improved stamina, flexibility, and strength.

Personal growth: Seniors may evaluate their success in restorative yoga by considering any personal development or changes they have gone through. They could, for instance, have become more self-aware or become more conscious and present in their everyday lives.

THE END